Soul Play

*A Workbook to Inspire and
Guide Your Soul Journey*

Soul Play

*A Workbook to
Inspire and Guide
Your Soul Journey*

PATRICIA GREER

A COMPANION VOLUME TO
BREAST CANCER: A SOUL JOURNEY

CHIRON PUBLICATIONS
ASHEVILLE, NORTH CAROLINA

© 2017 by Chiron Publications. All rights reserved. No part of this publication may be reproduced, stored in a retrieval system, or transmitted, in any form by any means, electronic, mechanical, photocopying, recording, or otherwise, without the prior written permission of the publisher, Chiron Publications, 932 Hendersonville Road, Suite 104, Asheville, North Carolina 28803.

www.ChironPublicatons.com

Interior and cover design by Cornelia G. Murariu.
Printed primarily in the United States of America.

ISBN 978-1-63051-423-5 paperback
ISBN 978-1-63051-424-2 hardcover
ISBN 978-1-63051-425-9 electronic
Library of Congress Cataloging-in-Publication Data

Names:	Greer, Patricia, 1940- author.
Title:	Soul play : a workbook to inspire and guide your soul journey / Patrica Greer.
Description:	Chiron Publications : Asheville, North Carolina, [2017]	"A companion volume to breast cancer: a soul journey."	Includes bibliographical references and index.
Identifiers:	LCCN 2017004892 (print)	LCCN 2017009549 (ebook)	ISBN 9781630514235 (paperback : alk. paper)	ISBN 9781630514242 (hardcover : alk. paper)	ISBN 9781630514259 (electronic)	ISBN 9781630514259 (E-book)
Subjects:	LCSH: Breast--Cancer--Patients--Rehabilitation.
Classification:	LCC RC280.B8 G7242 2017 (print)	LCC RC280.B8 (ebook)	DDC 616.99/449--dc23

LC record available at https://lccn.loc.gov/2017004892

In memory of my friend, Robin

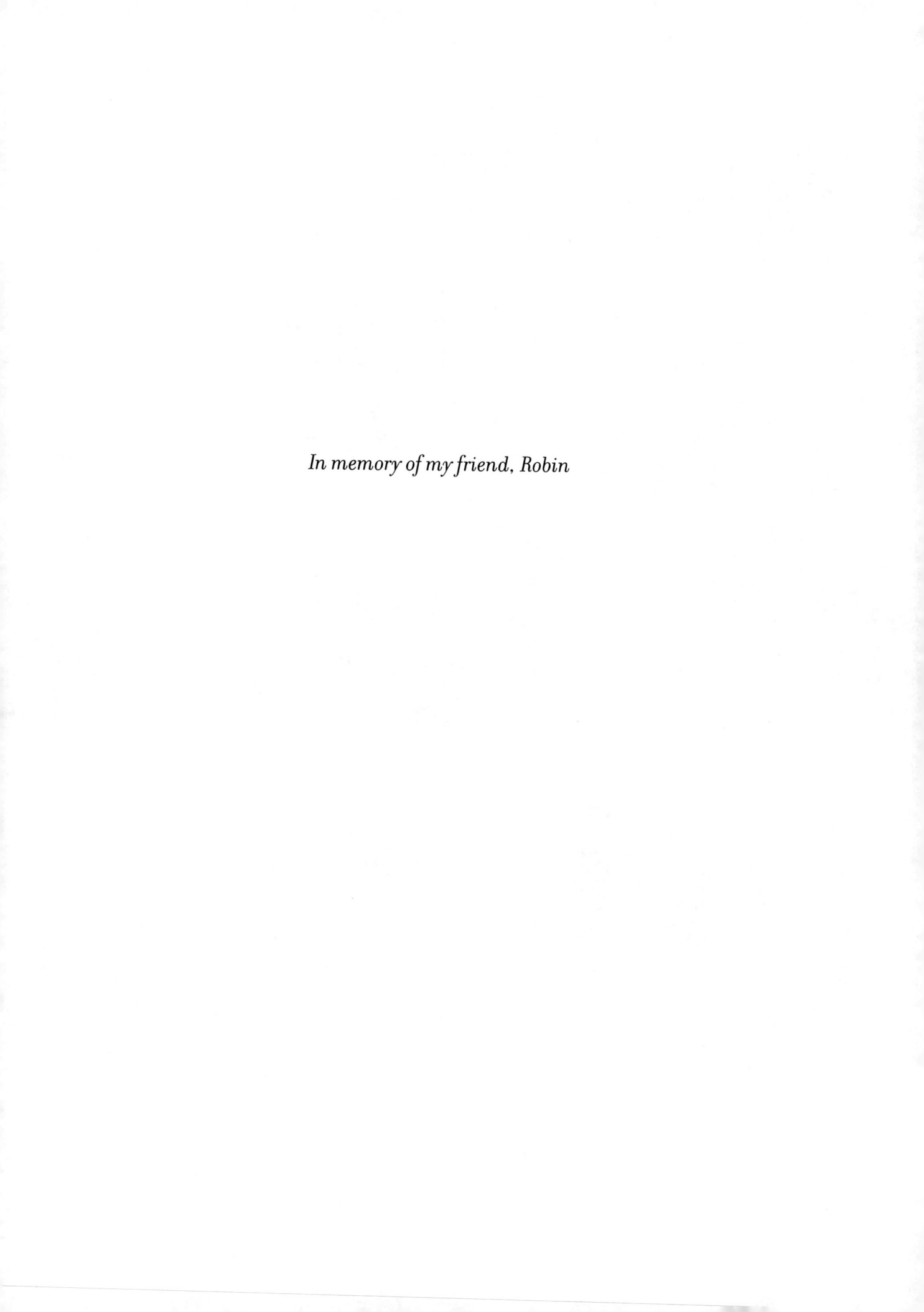

INTRODUCTION

I was asked by some women who read my book, *Breast Cancer: A Soul Journey*, if I would write a workbook to accompany it, offering thoughts and questions and reflections for women who want to go on their own soul journeys of exploration.

So here it is.

But I don't like the idea of a *work* book. It can sound like a chore, and many women with breast cancer don't want more work to do. Well, who does? I think it's more about a kind of play. Soul play, because soul loves to play, I believe. It's a serious and intense kind of play that may lead you to difficult truths, and it is definitely an important kind of psychological work. It is playing with words and thoughts and questions and images, which can take you to the depths of soul, that timeless, most authentic, truest part of yourself.

WHO MIGHT BENEFIT FROM THIS?

This exploration is for women who feel ready to look beneath the literal concerns of cancer – of which there are so many – and explore the inner insights and wisdom that may be embedded in their own experiences of illness. For some women, this may be early in treatment. For others, it may be months or years after diagnosis and treatment. I didn't write anything for a year after my diagnosis; I think I may have felt, perhaps unconsciously, that I needed all my energy to heal from the assault of the cancer. So you need to decide when, and if, this is a journey you feel called to take.

If you have read this far, you may be at least a little curious about the idea that cancer can be re-imagined as a soul journey. That can be a good place to start.

This path is not for everyone. Some women who have had cancer do not want to look back; they want to go forward, move on, put it behind them. You need to discern whether this journey of exploration is right for you. For those of you who do want to look back and look deeper, to embark upon your own soul journey, I offer these thoughts.

I had breast cancer, so that is the experience I worked with to move into the depths of soul. But it can be anything that propels you into looking at your life – any cancer, any illness, any crisis. If you have a different experience, just translate my words into the language of your life event.

The thoughts and suggestions in this guide are most useful if you first read my book *Breast Cancer: A Soul Journey,* because it tells one woman's story and reveals the power of journaling, poetry, and drawing to evoke the subtle dimensions of soul. Then, if you want to begin your own soul journey, use the ideas and questions on these pages to reflect and create your story.

This guide is, by its nature, only an introduction to a complex reality, only one possible map of the territory. It does not attempt to explain psychological issues or theories. Instead it offers you some ways of beginning to access some of the depths within yourself, of beginning to listen to, and honor, your own whispers of soul.

PART ONE

Some Ways of
Paying Attention to Soul

HOW TO BEGIN

It may begin with journaling, a practice of writing about . . . anything.

If you are new to journaling . . .

. . . you need paper and pencil or pen. Pretty simple. Some people love to search for a special, beautiful journal, something that would honor their thoughts and musings. But that has never worked for me – it always feels intimidating, like I have to come up with some Very Important and Meaningful Words and Ideas. I like an inexpensive spiral bound notebook, one that will fit in a large purse if I want to take it with me. Or a yellow legal pad where pages can be torn off and moved around. Or unlined computer paper for a looser arrangement of words or simple sketches. See what seems to appeal to your soul.

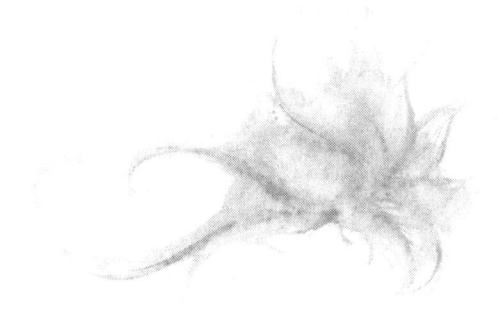

I think the work has to be a little messy, sometimes. It may not arrange itself in tidy paragraphs that progress clearly along a theme. Soul lurches and stumbles and circles back and down; you want to be able to erase and cross out and make changes as the mood strikes. Use whatever works for you. Experiment with different choices.

You may want to include some crayons or colored pencils or watercolors and maybe a simple art journal to contain your images. I think it is useful to date your entries and keep everything together and contained, however loosely, so that you can move forward and back through the entries as you wish. Maybe a notebook with a pocket to hold loose pages. Maybe just a large folder into which you can stuff all your musings and scraps of paper.

Though I call this a workbook, of sorts, I didn't want to make it the kind of book that has spaces for you to fill in after each idea. I don't think soul flourishes under that kind of restriction. Maybe your response will be several sentences or maybe it will be several pages. Maybe you will return to it at another day with some further musings. Let yourself wander in circles, if that feeds the process.

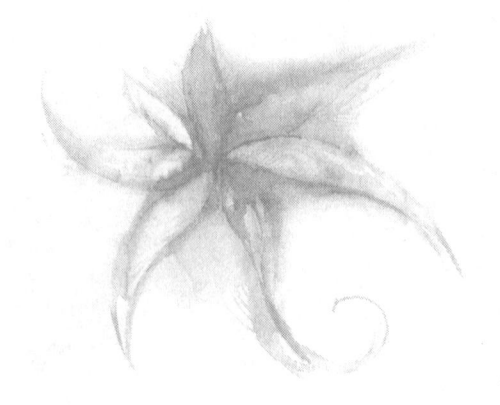

WHEN AND WHERE

So you have something to write with and something to write on. That was the simple part. Now all you need is time and a place. Not so simple.

Most women say they are busy, too busy. They say they are used to putting everyone else's needs before their own. So it may be a challenge to find time, and both the inner and outer space, to honor this process. You may have young children or a demanding career or both. If you are older and retired, you may have more free time, but it may still be difficult to take some of that time just for yourself. I have spoken to many women, young and old, who find it hard to justify doing something like this for themselves. They often feel that it is selfish or unnecessary. One woman told me she realized that the lack of personal and creative time in her life was impacting her physical health, but she just couldn't disappoint others in her life who wanted her attention.

I think the process begins by realizing that it is important, crucially important to your soul, to your deepest part of yourself.

And then, just start. Take the first step. And then another. See where it leads.

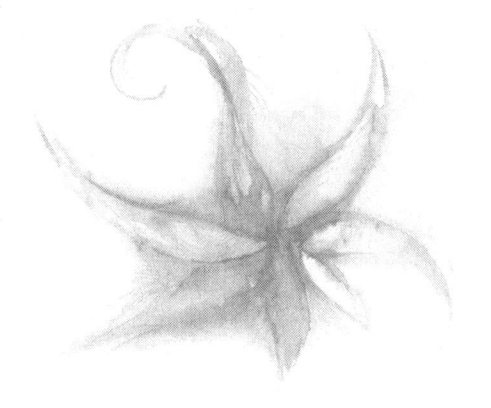

Find a rhythm that works for you.

You may decide this ahead of time or you may feel your way into it. Some people like to set a regular time to write, maybe early in the morning before the activities of the day start, or maybe in the evening when things have quieted down and there is some space for stillness. Some people find it works better to be less structured and write whenever and wherever they can. Perhaps you'll carry a small notebook with you and jot down some preliminary thoughts at your child's soccer game. Or maybe you'll go to a coffee shop and spend some time writing in the anonymity of the crowd. Or you may find that you like best to write in your garden in the summer, or pausing on a walk in the woods in the fall, or in your favorite chair in a room with a window to watch the weather in the winter.

Let soul lead you to the times and places that are most pleasing.

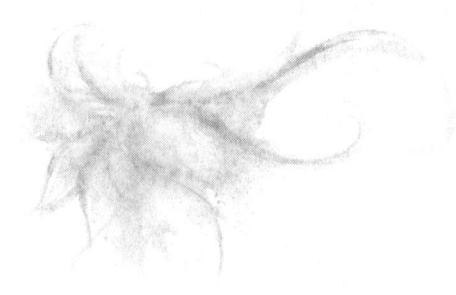

WHY

Why do this at all?

I think it is one of the best and easiest ways to give your soul space and place to express itself. It offers a way for you to connect more deeply to that part of you that I think of as soul, that mostly indefinable, ageless, deep inside place that is the truest you. By connecting to that deepest inner part of you, you may find that you are able to become more authentically and more fully who you are.

But you may still have some mixed feelings about the whole idea. Is this really worth it? Is it going to help anything? Might it cause change? Do you welcome such change?

You might stop right here and let the different parts of yourself speak. Take paper and pencil and begin with the voice that seems that loudest – what is it saying? Write it down. All of it.

Then pause for a while and see if there is another voice that wants to say something. Write it down.

Then pause again and see who wants to talk next. It may be another voice, or it may be the first voice wanting to answer. Allow the dialogue to go on until it feels finished and resolved.

Some parts of you may want change in your life; some parts may fear change. I think it's important to give attention to all your inner voices before you begin, or they may sabotage the process later. Hopefully you will come to an agreement that feels good enough and allows you to continue. If you still sense some resistance, you may promise to listen again later to the dissenting voices.

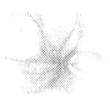

COLLECT QUOTES

You may want to have a separate section in your journal to collect quotes that are meaningful to you – a line of poetry, a thought from a favorite author, an idea from a movie or a play. Anything that catches your attention. You could spend a few minutes journaling about why it appeals to you, what you find important to remember. It might be a jumping off place for some of your own musings. Or you may just record it and return later to ponder its significance to you.

One of my favorite quotes, which I used in my book, is from the poet Anne Sexton:

"Put your ear down close to your soul and listen hard."

She captures so beautifully and directly what a soul journey is all about.

When you start collecting such ideas, you may find that some become signposts for your own journey, that they help to point the way and encourage your exploration.

Just collect whatever appeals to you. You can return later to ponder the significance and write more about how it impacts you.

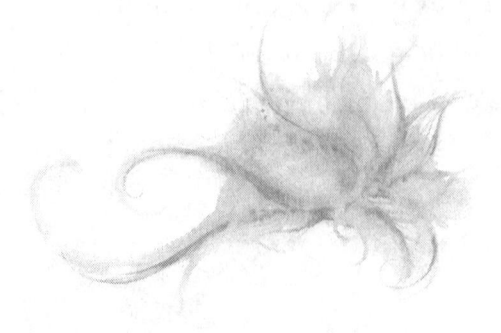

START WRITING

ACKNOWLEDGMENT OF GRATITUDE AND SADNESS

In my book, I began by acknowledging and thanking many people who walked with me on my journey and offered support along the way. You may want to call to mind and express gratitude to the people in your life who were there for you in your difficult moments, who offered words of encouragement or wordless caring. Summon their spirits in a circle with you and feel the energy and connection.

Go back in your life and remember the people who helped you become who you are. What are they like, what are their special gifts, what do you love about them? Fill your page and your heart with all the connections that sustained you along the way.

Some women have told me heart-breaking stories of friends who deserted them when they were diagnosed with cancer. Were these people unable to bear the anguish of a friend's pain? Did they not know what to say or do, and so found it easier to disappear? If there were people on your journey who disappointed you, who weren't able to walk with you, you may want to write about that hurt. Maybe you are able to forgive them, to free yourself of the energy drain on your psyche. Or maybe it's too soon, and you need to let yourself feel whatever you're feeling for as long as you feel it.

Write it all out. Eventually, you may be able to release the feelings and move on.

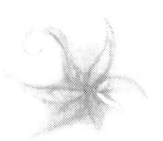

BEGIN WITH THE LITERAL STORY

When you set out to explore the teachings of your breast cancer experience, I think it is useful to start by writing about the literal story. Anything and everything you remember. It's a way of opening up the process, of letting the words start to flow. You may feel that you don't want to go back and remember the details of this painful time of your life, whether it was weeks or months or years ago.

You may wonder why? What's the point?

I think it helps to let yourself re-live some of the experience, even though it is painful, as a way of establishing a different relationship with cancer. It is something that happened to you, not of your choosing, not of your control. But it is something that you can choose to explore, that you can relate to, that you can plumb for wisdom. So this is a way of starting to make it conscious, to bring it into focus. Tell the stories.

Set aside some uninterrupted time when you can concentrate on one aspect of your story and write about it for a while. Get comfortable and quiet and give yourself enough time to feel that the recollection is complete.

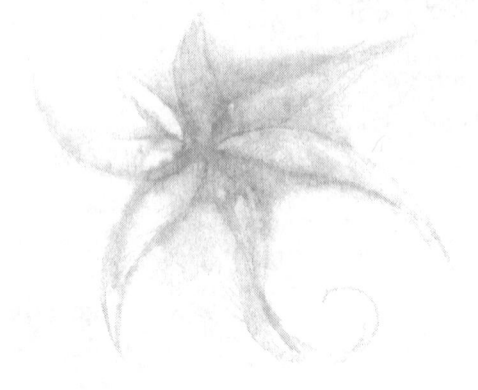

You might begin with some memories . . .

I recommend that you move slowly through the questions below, giving yourself time to linger over your response to each one. Perhaps as you engage in the process, remembering and writing, you may find that you recall more than you realized at first.

Where were you when you got the diagnosis? What time of day, what time of year?

Were you at home and got a phone call, as I was? What room were you in? What did it look like?

What had you been doing before the call came?

Were you out in public? What were you doing?

Were you at a doctor's office? What did the room look like, feel like? Who was with you?

What were your first thoughts and feelings? Did you have someone with you to talk to? Did you call someone to share the difficult news?

Use enough specific detail to carry yourself back to that time.

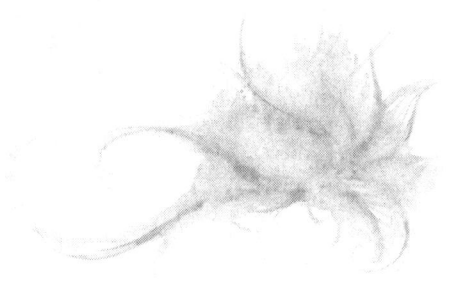

Then let the questions get larger. Where were you in your life when it happened? In your relationships? In your career? How were you spending your time?

How was it changed?

These are big questions, and they deserve some time to be answered. Sit with them for a while.

Go back and walk with yourself through the early days of the experience. What were your feelings? Panic? Disbelief? Fear? Anger? Confusion? Numbness? There may have been a mix of many feelings, so give yourself permission to linger here long enough to remember them all.

Even in the early onslaught of distress, were there any moments of faith or friendship or love that helped?

Do you remember a time when you felt compassion from someone on the medical team during your series of treatments? Maybe it was a touch, a glance, a word. Describe in detail where you were, who it was, what happened, how you felt.

If you were lucky, you had a good support system of friends and loved ones who helped you during the process. Recall some specific moments that touched you, and paint a word picture of each incident: the gift, the feelings, the bond. Maybe it was a time of tears, maybe a time of laughter. Maybe expressions of kindness and consolation. Maybe an unspoken connection. Take yourself back to that moment with words.

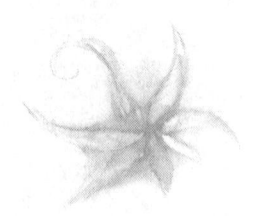

I suggest that you take your time with these recollections. They may bring up many strong feelings, so allow yourself to move slowly through the process.

When you went through treatments, surgery, chemotherapy and/or radiation, what was it like? Can you remember the first time – the details, the scene, the people, the feelings? Can you remember how you felt afterward, what you did?

What do you remember about your recovery time, where you were, what it was like? Was there one room where you tended to spend most of your time during the healing process? What did you like about it? Or dislike about it?

If you had chemotherapy, did you lose your hair? Let yourself write about the feelings. That is the hardest side effect for many women; was it for you? How did you cope with it? Could you sometimes laugh? Cry?

If you had surgery, do you remember the first time you looked at your scar? Your new body? The first time someone else looked at it?

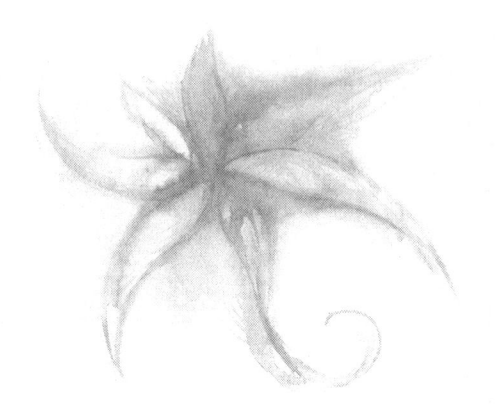

Have your feelings toward your body changed over time? Take some time to let yourself explore all your feelings, even if they are painful.

Can you be compassionate to yourself? How would you do this?

Can you see beauty and strength in your new body, even though it may not look exactly as it used to, as you may want it to?

Do you have any images associated with cancer or the treatment of cancer? Do you think of it as a battle? Do you think of the treatments that help to kill cancer cells as poison? Might you want to challenge that stance within yourself and come to a gentler acceptance of the life-giving help they provide?

Keep writing . . .

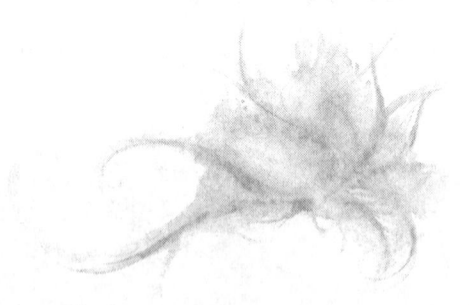

SINCE CANCER

I think of my life as *since* cancer now. Not *after* cancer. If you have had breast cancer, I think you know what I mean – I don't think we ever feel fully *after*. The fears of recurrence are always there, lurking. But for most of us, I think, there are changes in our lives since cancer. Maybe there are some that you think are better, maybe some that you think are worse. This exercise is a way of focusing your attention on all the changes, perhaps some that you have barely noticed. And it may give you an opportunity to include other changes that you want to make.

So just take a blank sheet of paper and begin a list.

Since cancer, I . . .

Just keep repeating the phrase and fill in an answer on each line.

Maybe you eat more kale or more chocolate.

Maybe you appreciate a beautiful sunrise or sunset more than ever. Or hate seeing them.

Maybe you feel more gratitude or more anger.

Maybe you don't rush as much. Maybe you rush more than ever.

Maybe you feel more patient with people, or yourself. Maybe less.

Just keep listing everything that occurs to you. Then pause, and list some more.

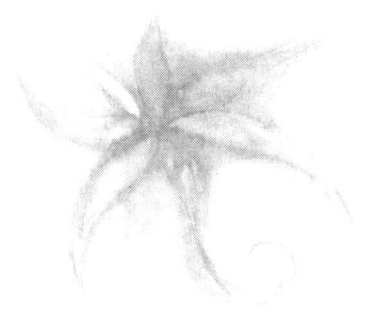

When you feel fully finished, take a look at the list. Analyze it.

Are there any changes that you feel are positive? Any that you feel are negative? Any that surprise you?

Are there any that you want to consciously try to increase or decrease? Sometimes we aren't even aware of changes that have occurred until we focus our attention on them. Are there areas of your life that you want to give more energy, so that they will increase? Or give less energy, so that they will decrease?

When you look over the entire list, what is your feeling? What would you say about the writer of this list? Be gentle with yourself, but honest.

If you were her best friend, is there any counsel you would offer her?

Support? Advice? Encouragement?

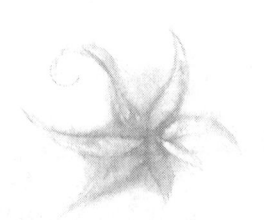

BEGIN TO MOVE AWAY FROM THE LITERAL: LOOSEN THE LANGUAGE

We usually write in sentences and paragraphs with one main thought or idea. The point of this exercise is just to begin to loosen your use of language a little. This more playful approach gives an opportunity for a less structured verbal expression, perhaps coming from another aspect of yourself. Maybe you will discover something new, something unexpected, something valuable.

So to begin, try playing with a *word picture*. Take a fairly large unlined piece of paper and start by putting a word in the center of it. You can use pencil or colors. For this exercise, you might want to start with the name of your illness as the central word. Then see what other words want to appear. Just write down any words that occur to you in any place on the paper, in any shape, in any arrangement.

Give yourself permission to take your time and have fun with this. Let yourself be surprised by what might want to appear on the page, as if you don't have to be in charge.

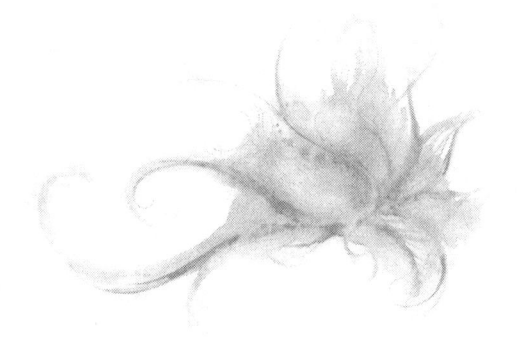

When you are finished, see what wanted to appear. Notice whether your words rushed onto the page or appeared slowly. Notice if they are in printing or cursive. Notice if they are different sizes. Notice if they connect and group in clusters or drop randomly onto the page. What do you associate to each of these possibilities?

If you used colors, what is your association to each one? Are some words in different colors? What might that suggest to you? Are there patterns of color? Do some colors touch, or overlap?

Write about each thing that you notice. Just feel your way into what the word picture may want to reveal to you.

Another time, try doing a word picture again, perhaps with a central word like:

    Soul

        Healing

            Balance

                Peace

                    Health

                        Joy

You will think of others.

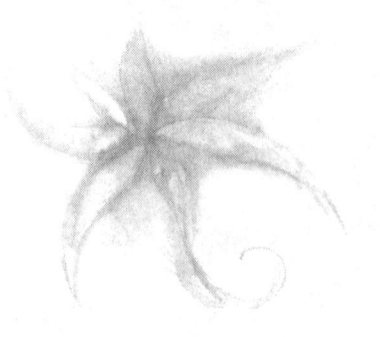

Next, try writing a poem. I know, you may say you don't do poetry, or you won't, or you don't even like to read it. But perhaps you could just suspend judgment and tell your inner critic to go off duty for a while and let you play. It's just to give your soul another way of letting it express itself.

The first version is writing a haiku, a very structured form of poetry consisting of 3 lines and a total of 17 syllables in the following arrangement: first line of 5 syllables, second line of 7 syllables, third line of 5 syllables. Because of its precise and detailed construction, it lends itself to focusing on one very specific image or thought. Maybe you could go outside and notice one aspect of nature that appeals to you. Maybe you could go within and look for one thought or feeling you want to express.

Here is an example of mine from when I was sitting outside last summer:

Bright flowers beckon,
Hummingbird comes to visit –
A summer blessing.

Try writing a haiku every day for a week or two. Just to see. Just to notice. Just to express. Are you looking at nature differently? Are you noticing your thoughts and feelings differently?

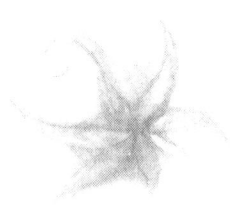

The second version is an unstructured poem. Let yourself focus on an idea or image and just allow the words to flow freely onto the page. Again, give up any thoughts of paragraphs and topic sentences and maybe even punctuation for now.

There are many examples of poetry scattered throughout my book. This is an excerpt from one poem that demonstrates the form and expresses some of my feelings about the benefits of writing:

I write to know.
It's as if I don't know
until the words come,
until the words tell me what I know.

It's not to remember, exactly,
it doesn't feel like that,
although somewhere I know
before words.

I write to see,
to take what's there, unformed,
and work it somehow,
feel it and work it
like clay in my hands
and make it appear
there
where I can see it.

Take some of your own clay and play with it a while and see what wants to happen.

When you have experimented with both versions of poetry, do you find that your soul prefers one way or the other? Does it enjoy the variety of both?

SEEK A SYMBOL

Or better yet, see what symbol may be seeking you, calling to you.

In your exploration of inner wisdom, it is important to open yourself to the pull of the symbolic world. If this is new to you, it may seem a bit strange, but, again, let the inner critic go for a walk. Away from you.

In my book, I wrote about my fascination with a glass box and how it summoned me to inner spaciousness before I had any understanding of what it meant. And I wrote about the meaning of a dream image of a redbud tree that called me back to writing as a way of connecting with soul.

Begin to notice if there is something that occasionally taps on the window of your consciousness and wants some attention. It may be a word, a piece of music, a dream image. It may be an object that you become aware of in a new way.

Have you been moved to collect shells or stones? Is there one in particular that seems to attract you?

Do you have a favorite art print that seems meaningful in some way?

Are you drawn to owls or eagles? A butterfly? A tree? A horse? Oceans? Stars?

If you look around for a while and don't detect anything, become more intentional in your search. Go outside into nature and look. Pay attention. See if you feel drawn to bring back some object from your wanderings.

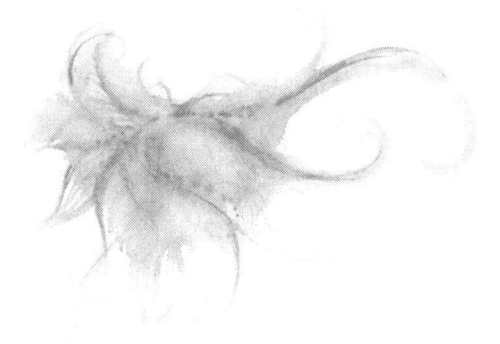

You may want to focus on the idea of finding something that represents your cancer to you. Not in a literal way, not a photo of someone who was supportive or the name of your oncologist or the wig you wore when you lost your hair. No. I want you to look for a looser, more subtle link. Take your time. Give your psyche time to mull and ponder and choose with discernment.

One symbol that related to cancer, for me, was a geode, a rock that has an interior space filled with crystal formations. Cancer was like that for me: ugly on the outside, with all the scars and treatments and side effects and fears. But inside, when I was finally able to look inside, there was treasure to be discovered . . . soul treasure.

Put your symbol where you can see it often, close to your writing space, if possible. Sit with it and let it permeate your thoughts and feelings.

Start to write about it . . . anything that comes to mind. For example, what is a tree? What is this particular tree like? What appeals to you or what repels you about this tree? What are your associations to it? Give yourself an expanse of time over days, weeks, months maybe, to connect to the object. What is the nature of this particular shell? What do you know about it? What do you see or think of when you look at it? How is it different from other shells?

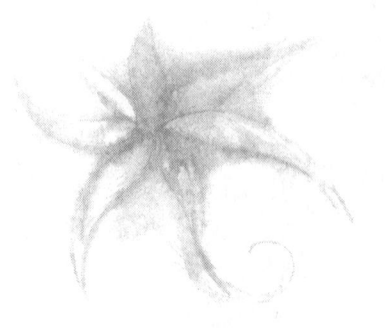

Gradually, instead of just writing about the object, start letting it speak to you.

What do I mean by that?

Again, suspend judgment, if you can, and just sink into a quiet space where you can listen to hear if the stone or the flower or the butterfly has something to teach you. Not that a stone or a butterfly can talk or that you will hear voices. Rather, it is that in the relationship with the object, whatever drew you to it, there may be a lesson for you. You might ask it what it has to teach you, what it wants you to know. Just ask it, and wait for an answer. Expect it. Welcome it. Thank it.

In your writing, you will discover why you felt drawn, for instance, to an owl. What is it about an owl that attracts you and holds meaning for you? What might owl-ness have to teach you about your life?

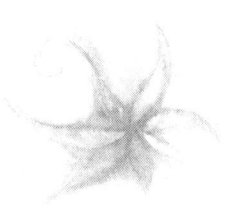

DREAM WORK

Dreams are one of the most available ways of linking to the unconscious because we all dream every night. But we don't always remember our dreams. And we don't always think they are important. I believe that they are. And maybe if you do some work with them, play with them, you will too. I describe several dreams in my book and demonstrate ways of thinking about their meanings in my life.

If you don't often remember your dreams, you might want to be more deliberate about capturing them. You can set an intention before you go to sleep that you want to remember your dreams that night. Put paper and pencil close to your bed and as soon as you wake up, write down all that you remember about the dream you had. If you wait until you get into the busyness of your day, much of the dream world may be forgotten.

I believe that dreams often come to tell us about something that we are not paying attention to, to adjust something in our vision of ourselves, our lives, our world. This means that the dream may be suggesting a kind of course correction. We see things, ourselves included, in a limited way – the way of an ego position. We may see ourselves as we want to be seen, or we may see ourselves in a limited way that doesn't recognize the full array of choices available to us. Dreams offer a deeper and wider perspective. You may want to begin to pay attention to new possibilities that present themselves.

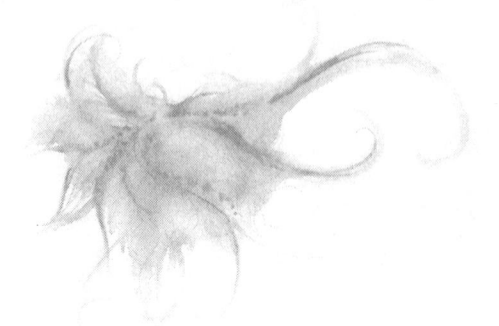

Dream work is rich and complicated. It is always helpful, I think, to work with a therapist to plumb the depths of unconscious meanings. But I also think that you can begin to access much meaning from a dream by working with it yourself. These suggestions offer a way to begin to value and understand what dreams may want to teach us.

You can work with the dream in much the same way as the objects you found. You might begin by reading the dream out loud, maybe a couple of times. See if there are any more details that come to mind as you give voice to the dream, and write those down as well.

Then note each person, each animal, each object in your dream and write down your associations to each one. I sometimes suggest, as a way of starting, to imagine that you are talking to someone who doesn't know the meaning of the word you are using. What is a lion? What is a mountain? That gives you a general start.

Then think about what lion or mountain means to you. Are lions frightening? Majestic? Predatory killers? Fierce? Is a mountain a place where you love to ski? Something to climb? A place to get a higher view of things? A frightening place? After you have exhausted your personal meanings and associations, you may want to consider cultural meanings from sources like myths, stories, art, religion.

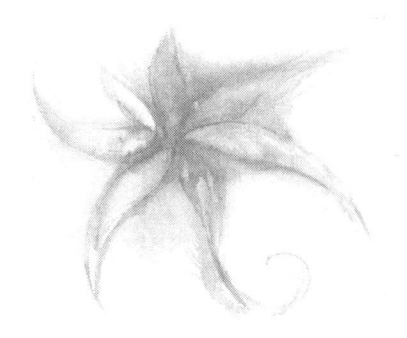

If there are people in your dream, describe their main characteristics in a few words.

Is this someone with whom you have a close, current relationship? If so, the dream may be trying to tell you something about that relationship. But often the person is unexpected: I frequently hear dreamers say, "I can't imagine why he or she would be in my dream."

Most dream theorists believe that usually everything in your dream is a part of you. When you think of the description of the person, does some part of it resonate with you? Can you see yourself in that portrayal? If you can't see any similarities at first, look more closely. Notice what you particularly like or dislike about the person, and then see if those qualities may be in you.

Give yourself time to ponder this. Sometimes we don't want to see in ourselves the traits that we may all too easily see and criticize in someone else.

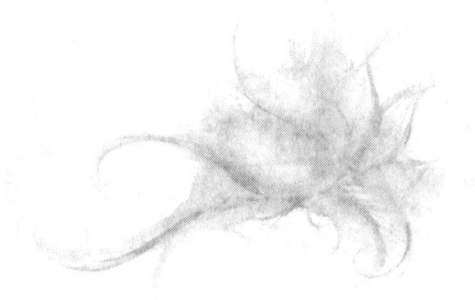

What is the setting of the dream? Is it familiar to you? Is it from a particular time in your life? What was going on at that time? What is your reaction to the place?

Pay attention to the language of dreams – puns, double meanings, subtleties.

Pay attention to the overall feeling that you have about the dream.

Pay attention to the particularity of the image. It is this kind of dog, with these characteristics, in this situation, demonstrating this behavior. Write about it all, and see what emerges.

Then try to understand the dream in the context of your life. Dreams often use what we call "day residue," something that happened in waking life that day. Usually, though, the message goes beyond a simple retelling of an event or situation. What is the theme of the dream? Is there some place in your life where you experience that theme? So, for example, if you are in dangerous circumstances in the dream, is there something that you experience as dangerous in your waking life?

Another thing you might do is draw an image from a dream. As I share in my book, when I drew a tree that had appeared in a dream, I saw things about it that I hadn't been aware of. The trunk was actually severed in one place and had grown sideways for a while. I was then able to associate to the particular details of the tree trunk that came to have meaning for me.

This is a brief introduction to the rich and layered complexity of dream work, but my hope is that it is enough to get you interested, if you haven't been, and to get you started on the exploration of your own fruitful dream world.

DIALOGUE WITH INNER FIGURES

Yes, you have them, I believe. I think we all have inner wisdom figures that may help us in this journey of soul. In my book, I describe interactions with an inner female figure named Soul Woman. I might have wished for a more subtle or more sophisticated name, but that's the one she seemed to choose. In many ways, she was not as I might have imagined her, and that confirmed for me that she had come to teach me something beyond what I thought I knew. She led me to value feminine consciousness and strength in myself and in the world in new ways I deeply appreciate.

How to access such an inner figure? It may be a figure from a dream or it may be one that you deliberately summon and ask for help. Begin by creating a quiet time and place for yourself to engage for a while in this communication. Let yourself settle into stillness and rest there for a while. Then you may want to ask that a figure appears to help you in some way.

Maybe you have a specific question. Maybe you want to know what cancer may be able to teach you. Maybe you want to consider making adjustments in your life.

And then you wait. And wait. It may take a while, and you may find yourself getting impatient, and perhaps that is part of your lesson. Maybe no figure will appear the first time you do this. I think you have to trust the process and accept whatever teaching comes.

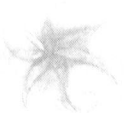

If you have a meeting with an inner figure, it is important to write about the experience. You may want to write the questions and responses during the process, or you may want to wait until it feels finished and then write about what transpired. I think it's important to express gratitude to the figure that came to you when it is over, just as you would to an outer world figure.

How do we understand such meetings? I think that we are all much more complex than our small ego-bound selves, and that we can access deeper parts of ourselves if we are intentional about it. You may think of this as prayer and spirit and inspiration; I think there are many languages and words that may describe the same thing, and may get us to the same reality. I think the important thing is that we get there, that we respect the teaching and the teacher, that we feel gratitude.

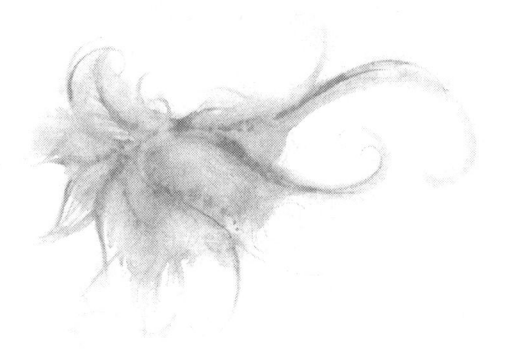

DRAWING/ART JOURNAL

Another way of accessing and tracking the inner world is through art work. I'm not talking about painting a pretty picture or trying to accurately reproduce a pewter pitcher with all the proper shading and shadow. This is about tapping into the shading and shadow in yourself, in your inner world.

To begin, you need paper and color. If this is new for you, you may want to keep it simple. The easiest choices are colored pencils, crayons, or markers, but you could also try pastels, watercolors, or acrylics. Or even finger paint.

I think that abstract work affords the best expression of inner reality. Act first, think later. Just let colors and shapes occur on the paper in any way they seem to want to. Let yourself experiment and see what appears.

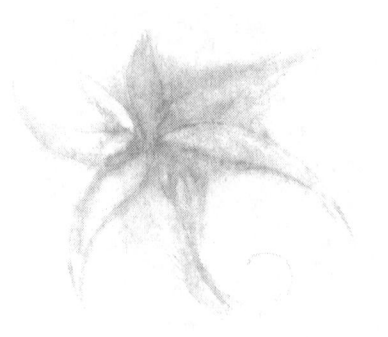

When it feels finished, look at it and write about it. What does each particular color make you feel? What about the shapes interest you? What do the patterns of lines and swirls suggest to you?

Where is the energy in the drawing? How is it moving or where is it blocked? Can you, for instance, feel such an energy flow or blockage in your body?

Some people like to do regular journaling with shapes and colors instead of words. One idea is to begin each art journal session by drawing a large circle on the page and then letting color and form appear within it – a way of containing the material in a simplified version of the complex mandala drawings that are currently popular. When you feel finished, ask yourself the same questions. In this version, you may notice that parts of the drawing extend outside the boundaries of the circle. How does that feel? What do you associate to it?

Experiment with what appeals to you and what seems to yield the richest images for contemplation.

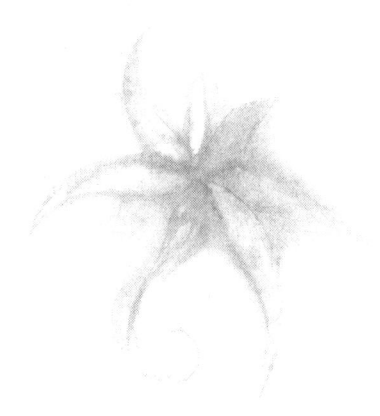

PART TWO

Themes from the Book
Breast Cancer: A Soul Journey

Now that you've spent some time working with ways of accessing soul in Part One, Part Two offers you specific reflections and questions based on the chapters and interludes of poetry in my book, *Breast Cancer: A Soul Journey*. It is best used, I think, by first reading the entire book to get a sense of the overall journey, and then by re-reading each part of the book that pertains to each set of themes. The chapters are short, so they are easy to re-read before exploring each group of ideas. Some may speak to you more than others, but you may want to spend a little time with all of them to see if your soul wants to respond.

I would suggest reading and working with one thought at a time, to give yourself a chance to deepen into your own experience and personal meaning. Write about your responses and allow time to reflect and add and change. If you feel called to write a poem or draw a picture or dance a response, give your soul permission to reply in any way that it wants.

You may, of course, skip any that don't appeal to you. But a word of caution. Ego does not like to be challenged. At all. Perhaps the area that seems unimportant or unappealing to you may be the most valuable for you to consider. Perhaps the question that you want to ignore is the most important one for you to work with. Perhaps the very thing that you want to avoid is the thing that you are avoiding in your life, that you should take a look at.

CHAPTER ONE
METAPHOR AND MEANING

The idea of metaphor, words that connect to an idea in a non-literal way, can begin to take you to deeper realms of meaning, to begin to excavate beneath the objective reality. Is there an image that speaks to your experience of cancer? For me, a painting captured some of the complexity of my experience and feelings. As I describe in the book, the gentle movements of blues and greens are slashed through and torn apart – exactly how my life felt when I got the diagnosis.

Is there a painting that you think of? A sculpture, a poem, a piece of music, a dance, an aspect of nature? What about it relates to your illness? How does it amplify your experience and help you to deepen into it? Settle in for a while.

Are there words from other writers, perhaps, that resonate with your experience? You might want to leave pages in your journal to collect some as you come across them. Once you start looking, you may find more than you expected.

Most women have many fears about breast cancer: fear of treatments, of side effects, of disfigurement or loss of a breast, and ultimately of death. What were and are your specific fears?

What were your sources of strength that helped you get through the challenges?

How do you hold the ongoing fear of recurrence? The fear of death? How often do you think of these fears? How do they affect your life? For me, the fear of death is real and scary, but it also makes me feel more grateful for the small joys of life, more appreciative of each day. Is this true in any way for you?

I speak of illness as a possible call to evaluate and make changes in one's life. This is not an accusation of you having done anything wrong to cause your illness. In fact, it is not about cause at all. But it can be an opportunity to take stock and look at possible adjustments in perspective or values or priorities. Can you begin to consider that cancer might provide such an opening for you?

I found I needed a sense of inner sanctuary, a sense of clearing out inner space to have time to listen to the longings of soul. Do you experience anything like that? Do you honor it? How? Are there other things you could do? Are there other things you feel called to do?

Breast cancer is overwhelmingly a woman's disease. This might be a time to consider your relationships with other women in your life. It might be a time to consider your relationship with the inner feminine, that aspect of yourself that honors feminine values. What are those values in your life? Is your life aligned with those priorities?

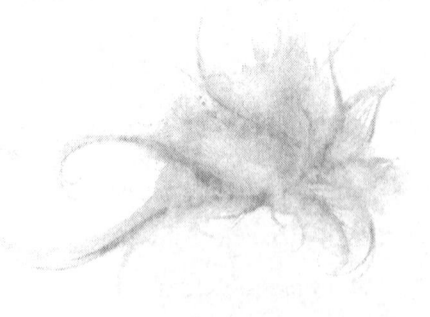

INTERLUDE: SPEAKING OF FAIRY GODMOTHERS

I used the ancient fairy tale of *Sleeping Beauty* to express some of my concerns about what I/we may be ignoring in our lives.

What are you neglecting in your life?

What are you valuing in your life that may not be feeding your soul?

Are you sleeping through parts of your life?

Has the battle with cancer awakened you to any more essential truths of your life?

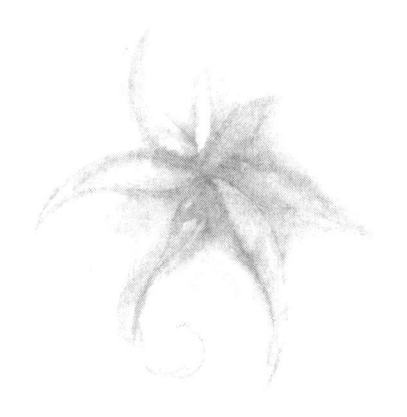

CHAPTER TWO
A VISION OF SOUL

Ego is the more limited part of ourselves, mostly conscious, that likes to be in charge and believes that it is. Psyche is the more complete part of ourselves that includes unconscious elements, that sometimes challenges ego's stance.

Imagine and write out a dialogue between ego and psyche and let them discuss some issue that is current with you. When you give psyche equal air time, are there new ideas that are presented to you?

Individuation is becoming more fully oneself. Is that a conscious goal for you? How do you embrace that in your life?

Are there parts of you that may not want individuation, that may be sabotaging your efforts? Give them a chance to speak again.

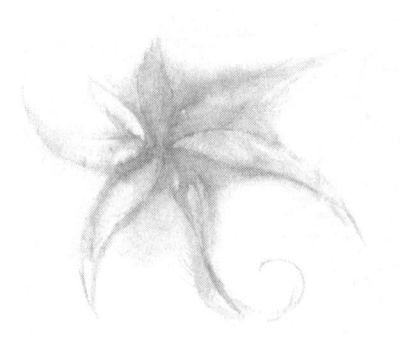

This chapter introduces a dream and demonstrates some ways of working with it. If you have been keeping a dream journal, you might want to select a recent dream and begin to work with it in the ways described earlier.

In my book, I describe my cancer as the lump around which my soul grew – like the irritation in a mollusk around which a pearl grows. Did you experience anything like that?

I think of soul as the deepest, truest part of myself, that ageless part that is most essentially me. What is the meaning of soul for you? Can you describe it? Are there writers, poets, philosophers, theologians whose definition of soul speak to you? You may want to save some pages in your journal to collect more quotes and examples. Let your soul choose.

What does your soul want? Where do you feel its pull in your life? Do you respond? Give yourself some time to linger here and write.

For me, it is most often poetry that calls me to soul. For others it may be classical music, jazz, ballet, painting, working with clay, gardening, yoga, meditation.

What is it for you? How do you honor it? Are you perhaps called to try an additional path?

How does your soul like to play? How do you honor the creativity that feeds soul?

One of the ways that I like is photography, especially nature photography. It gets me outside into the healing context of nature and it slows me down. I pause. I notice more, even the smallest flower or a dewdrop on a leaf. A sunset. A branch made magical with ice on it. Fog covering a lake in early morning. A red bird silhouetted against dark branches. I pause, I notice, I savor, and I feel gratitude.

How do you find a way to pause from your busyness and give time to your soul?

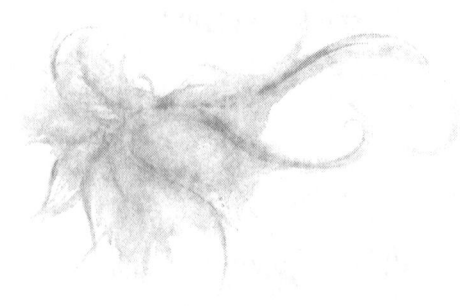

INTERLUDE: SOUL PLAY

How does your life seesaw between control and chaos? Is your life too chaotic? Or not chaotic enough?

Do you try to control too much? Are you afraid of losing control, letting go? Do you need to have more control in your life?

Do you seek balance? Are you able, at least some of the time, to find it?

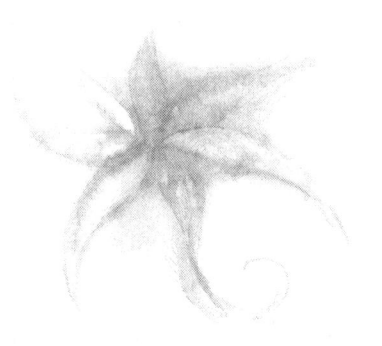

CHAPTER THREE
A VIEW OF FEMININE CONSCIOUSNESS

Have you been drawn to an image or an activity that may express your soul's desire? What is your soul longing for? How do you let it tell you what it wants?

In your busyness, are you sometimes called to slow down, to be quiet, to observe, to appreciate, to give gratitude? How do you restore and replenish your energy?

In the external world, do you ever feel burdened by disorder, by too much stuff? Can you clear out some of the clutter? Organize? Simplify? Pare down to essentials? If you do this, do you feel lighter? More free? Do you feel more inner space opening up to give you room to be still and peaceful?

Sometimes we rush to fill the inner emptiness because we feel afraid of it. I write about the woman who needs to eat or drink or shop to fill the emptiness inside. Do you rush to fill an emptiness with things that don't really nourish? Can you imagine letting go of any of those quick fixes and instead making a choice that is more deeply satisfying, more nurturing to your soul?

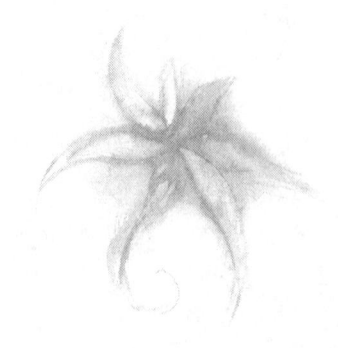

Do you ever feel that you are playing a series of roles in your life, roles that are mostly determined by others? Do you feel a longing to discover who you are at your deepest essence?

What are some titles that you would give to the roles you play?

What are some words that you would use to describe your authentic self?

Perhaps put them side by side and see how they compare. If you weren't afraid, how would you begin to make changes to become closer to your authentic self?

Are there women in your life or characters from books or movies that carry a sense of authenticity for you? Take time to describe each one. What about her appeals to you? How does she seem to be her own person? How might she inspire you to seek more authenticity for yourself?

Can you make some time in your busy schedule for small retreats, for time to be with yourself? What would you commit to do, as a way of starting the process? When? How often? What would you use as a way to deepen into yourself – meditation, journaling, art work, time in nature? What appeals to your soul?

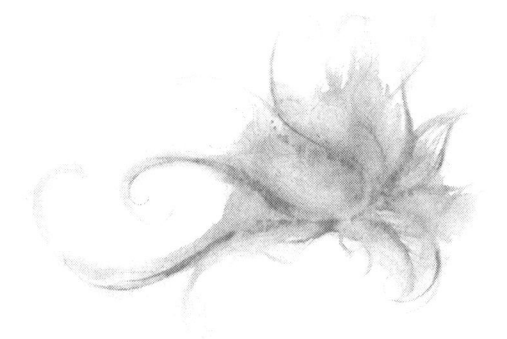

INTERLUDE: THE SEDUCTION OF ORDER

Is order a strong ruling force in your life?

When life is messy, do you fight it? Do you tolerate it? Do you embrace it? Do you learn from it?

Cancer certainly interrupts the life we intended to have. How have you dealt with the disruption?

Has cancer changed the course of your life in meaningful ways? Do you have a new relationship with order?

With soul?

With life?

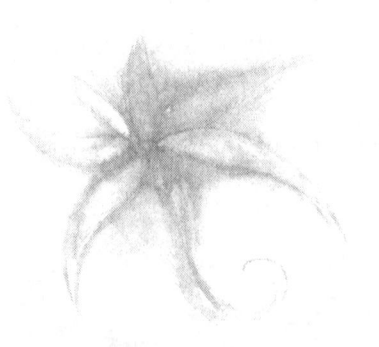

CHAPTER FOUR
SYMPTOM AND SYMBOL

A physical symptom may call attention to an area of *dis-ease* in your life. I don't mean in a causal way, but in a symbolic way.

Meditate on your particular illness and see if it connects to some place in your life that you may want to change.

Has your illness been a wake-up call for you? In what ways?

For many women, the loss of hair from chemotherapy is one of the most difficult realities to endure. What was your experience? Go back and recall the details.

Did you get a wig? Did you wear scarves? Did you appear in public without disguising your baldness? How did people react, loved ones, friends, strangers? How did you feel?

As you write about your hair and its loss, what are some meanings for you, literal and symbolic? What does hair mean to you? How important is it?

If you had breast cancer, what are your associations to the site of the tumor? Let yourself write about possible connections to breast for you. Nurturing and being nurtured? Giving and receiving? Mother/child issues? Sexuality? Femininity? Do any of these associations lead you to issues in your life that you want to ponder?

I wrote about the healing power of nature for me. This isn't about curing the cancer, but rather is a sense of possible healing in my life, a kind of balm for my soul. Where do you find such healing?

In this chapter, I describe an experience of meeting with an inner figure who became a teacher for me. I shared earlier, in Part One, how you might summon such a figure to help you. Experiment with accessing an inner part of yourself that connects to cancer in some way for you. Describe the figure in detail. What are your feelings about him/her/it? Are you surprised by any aspects?

Describe the circumstances of the meeting. A familiar place? Outside or inside? Any associations?

What are the implications for your life? That's a big question – give yourself time to consider it carefully.

This is an important technique that you may want to use again to access inner guidance and wisdom. Always evaluate the teaching that you receive and decide if it is something that you think is useful, that you think might be an important insight for your life. If so, write about ways that you might begin to implement changes that you want to make.

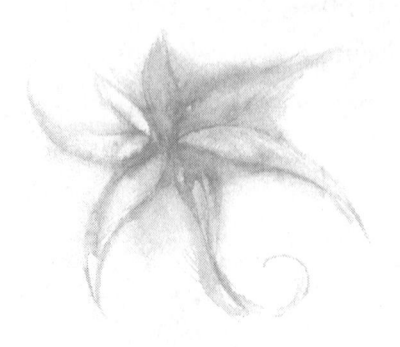

INTERLUDE: THE CANCER OF SILENCE

Have you experienced being silenced by someone? By a group of others? By society in general?

Do you sometimes silence yourself? Why?

Write about some specific times that you didn't give voice to something you thought or felt. How did you feel about it? If you could go back, would you want to do something different? What do you imagine it would have felt like to speak your truth?

Have you also experienced silence as a gift, chosen intentionally to honor your soul? Describe how you experience this silence. What are its rewards?

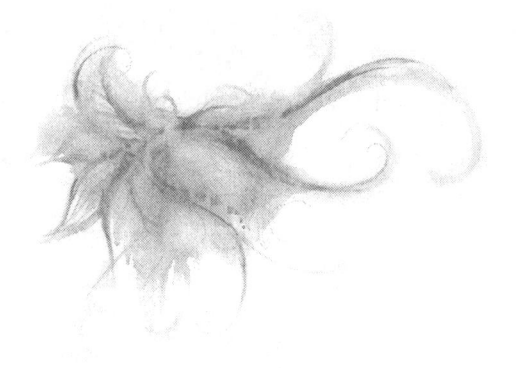

CHAPTER FIVE
IMAGES OF SELF

What is an image of your cancer? Write about it in prose or in poetry. Draw it. Color it. Paint it. Dance it. Find a symbol of it and write about the layers of meaning.

Is there a way that your experience of cancer connects with your sense of Self?

What are some images that come to mind when you think about your experience of cancer? Is there a dream, recent or remembered, that seems to connect with cancer or Self in some way? Work with it.

Draw an image from a dream that you remember. Is there anything unexpected in the drawing? What might it have to teach you?

For me, the image of tree became a strong connection to Self. What is yours?

What are your associations, connections, meanings?

What are possible messages for you? What are you learning from it?

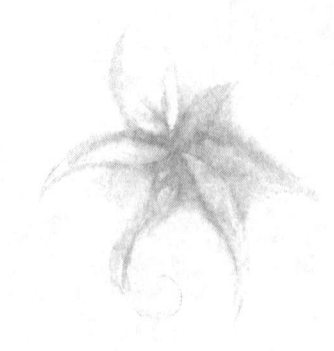

INTERLUDE: THE WEB

Let your inner poet play with an image of meaning, of connection. What patterns and images appear on the page? How does it want to flow?

Imagine a symbol that suggests connectedness to you. Perhaps the rings of a tree. Perhaps the root system of a plant. Perhaps the whorls of a shell. What comes to mind?

Imagine yourself as a tree. What do you feel?

Imagine yourself on a circular staircase. Are you going up or down? What do you see and hear? How does it feel to move yourself in circles?

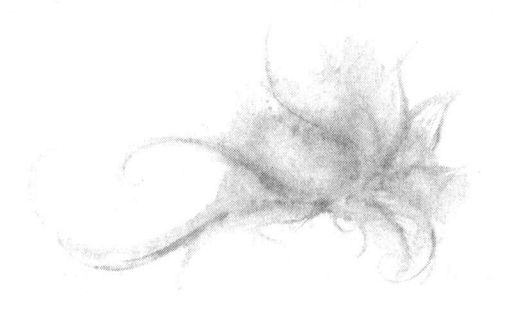

CHAPTER SIX
THE TEMPLE OF WOMEN

This chapter contains another active imagination experience with my inner figure, Soul Woman. For me, some of the teachings came in a wordless exchange, valuing silence and simplicity.

If you have had an experience with an inner figure, you might want to ask for another meeting. Pay attention to all the details beyond the exchange of words and see if there are messages there as well.

Try to find ways to amplify the experience, to honor it, to turn up the volume so you can hear the message more clearly. You might draw or paint a picture. You might work with clay. You might create and do a dance. You might find an object that carries the meaning for you.

In my book, I describe the process of sandplay, which is a Jungian technique of choosing and arranging objects in a pattern that can yield meaning. You might take some of the objects you have collected and place them on a table top or other flat surface. See if there are any connections that are suggested by the way you place them.

Some of the themes that emerged for me were centered on patriarchal privilege and feminine strength. Although I find that many of my issues are shared by other women, your experience may lead to very different insights. The content is specific to each woman, but the process may be similar for all of us. I share my soul journey as one example of a way to access the inner wisdom that may become available through an exploration of illness or crisis.

Spend some time discerning some messages that are relevant to your life. Allow yourself time to linger here and plan to come back and revisit these questions again.

INTERLUDE: WORDING THE PROCESS

For me, writing is an important way of connecting to my deeper self, my soul.

What are some ways that work for you? Write about how it works for you, how you forge a relationship to your soul.

Are you faithful to your process?

Are there ways you might go deeper?

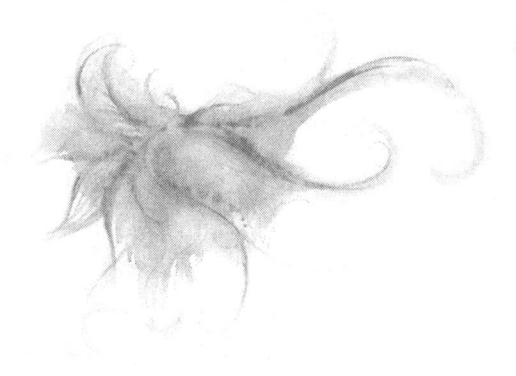

CHAPTER SEVEN
A BLAZE FOR THE JOURNEY

Spend some time thinking about and describing some possible growing edges in your life. What might you want to do if you were not afraid to try? What is calling to you?

How do you experience conflicts within yourself about being and having?

How does consumerism play a role in your life? How does it relate to your self-identity? Your self-worth?

How do you understand inner poverty, inner simplicity? Is it a value for you? If so, how do you honor it in your life?

Are you finding ways in your life to make a *giveaway,* a gift of yourself that is freely given to others?

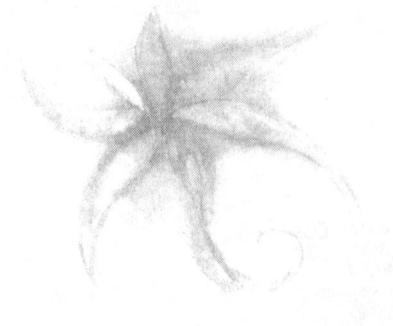

INTERLUDE: RICH

I wrote about the differences I felt among different kind of riches: superficial, ornamental riches compared with the idea of *richness* and *rich,* suggestive of a more spiritual nature. What are your associations to the differences?

What are some words you would choose that suggest a contrast between superficial values and values that are more authentic and meaningful?

Where do you see those differences playing out in your life?

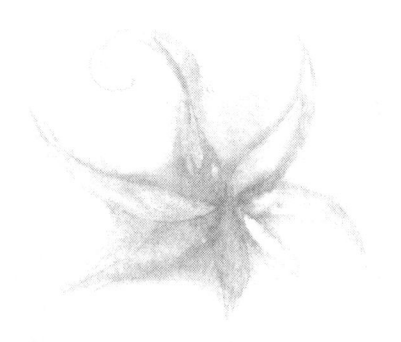

CHAPTER EIGHT
THE JOURNEY CONTINUES

Do you have lingering fears that continue to distress you since your experience of cancer? What are they?

What are the lessons you have taken away from your experience of serious illness? Do you feel that you are faithful to them?

Do you distinguish between process and product in your life? Do you focus on one to the detriment of the other? Have you found any resolution in the conflict?

One of the lessons I learned from illness is giving myself permission to rest. I know that I need to find ways to let my body find respite. Have you learned of its importance? Do you honor it in your life?

One of the most important pieces of advice that I give to friends who are going through the ordeal of serious illness is "be gentle with yourself." Are you able to do that?

What advice would you give to a friend or to yourself?

Are you able to savor the present moment of life? Do you ever experience conflict, as I did, between efficiency on one side and leisure and joy on the other? How do you deal with it?

Do you feel any difficulty in balancing a desire for external relationships on the one hand and a yearning for an inner relationship with your deeper self, your soul? How do you honor both? What are the factors that determine your choices when they need to be made? Do they feel authentic?

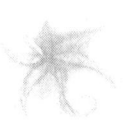

INTERLUDE: DECEMBER

For me, the month of December, a time of preparation for and celebration of Christmas, presents a tension between the spiritual and the material. Do you share a similar feeling? How does it manifest in your life? How do you try to resolve it?

What other situation might represent such a struggle in your life? Is it a time of year, a certain situation, a relationship? Write about the details of the dilemma, your feelings, your struggles.

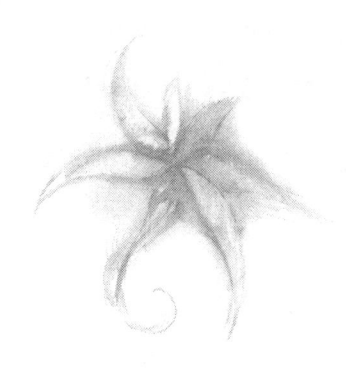

LAST CHAPTER
FINAL THOUGHTS

What are your final thoughts about your experience with cancer? You might want to look back over what you have written and explored, and see what themes emerge.

Cancer is a brutal disease, a difficult journey. It is a path never chosen, but for many of us, it is the path that must be travelled. There are losses, to be sure. But are there also any gifts that may be gained from the experience?

Have you changed, since cancer, in any ways that bring more peace? More appreciation? More connection? More depth?

Have you found ways to give back to the world, to find something meaningful to do?

Are you using your gifts of creativity?

Is there something you want to challenge yourself to do?

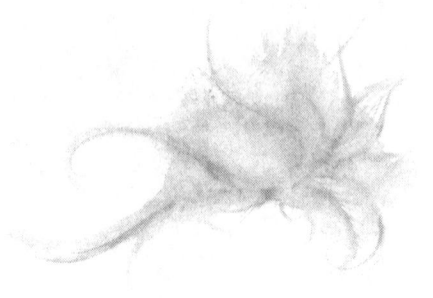

Since cancer, I often challenge myself with several questions.

Have I learned enough?

Have I done enough?

Have I been courageous enough?

Have I spoken and lived my truth?

Have I loved well enough?

How would you answer these questions? What other questions occur to you? Is there a daily practice that you may want to begin to include in your life since cancer?

As you come to the end of this process, know that you are at the beginning of another. And then another. And then …

Will you give yourself permission to continue? Will you give yourself time to continue?

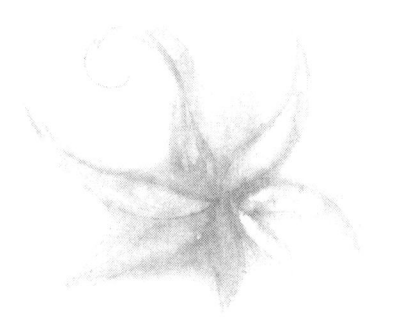

My hope for you is that through this journey you have connected with yourself at a deeper and more authentic level, that you have explored your inner world and value the experience.

My wish for you is that you make a promise to yourself: to continue to find ways to listen to the whispers of soul and to honor them in your life.

May your journey be rich
and meaningful.
Not easy —
easy is not the point.

May you learn much
and be certain of little,
allowing yourself to walk a path
that sometimes has no footprints
ahead of yours.

Keep going.
The rules are simple, I think:
notice,
care,
appreciate.

Go slow sometimes
so you can go deep.
Seek
and savor.

Find what is yours to do in the world,
the exact dead-center place
that uses all of you.
And then do it.

CPSIA information can be obtained
at www.ICGtesting.com
Printed in the USA
FFOW01n0232160517
35596FF